This book is dedicated to the *classic* individuals who paved the way, step by step.

Copyright © 2019 by Latonya D. Hughes

All rights reserved. No part of this book may be reproduced or used in any manner without written permission of the copyright owner except for the use of quotations in a book review. For more information, address: www.leadhq.care

FIRST EDITION

Leading

with

CLASS

Intentionally

The 21 Steps

A GIFT BOOK

Edited by Nara Y. Hughes

Personal Reflections

The Seat

The Team

The Respondent

The Replacement

The Line

The Concerned

The Moment

The Seat

As I *intentionally* walked into the conference room, all of the seats were taken, except for the one at the head of the table. As expected, I knew that seat was saved for me. Well, as I proceeded to sit down, one of the managers entered the room and stated,

"You're in my seat".

I quickly replied, "Oh! My apology". I took a quick look around the room, noticing all the seats were taken. Twenty people in the room and not a vacant seat. I was the newbie, the one they all reported too, but I did not have a seat. But did I need one?

Step #1

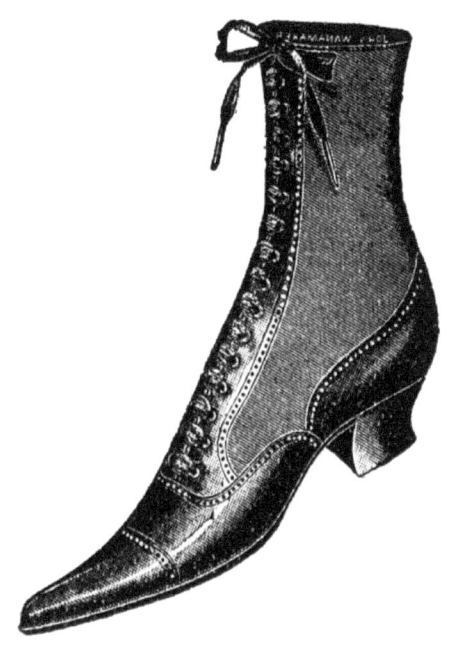

Sit down!

Should the leader sit at the head of the table? Maybe the leader should sit among the people. It's not the location of seat that determines power.

Step #2

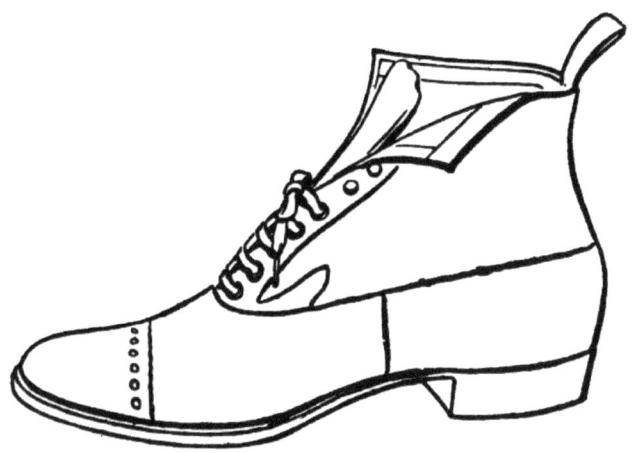

Identify who's leading.

The informal leader has taken on the role of leading the others, since leadership changes are frequently occurring.

Step #3

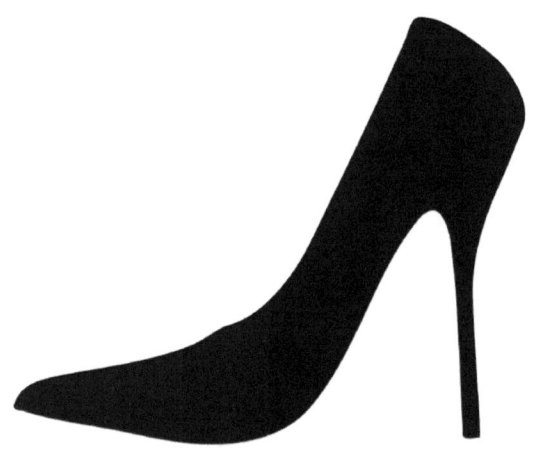

Ask for thoughts.

Who are the informal leaders? These are the people who typically don't have much to say, but are very observant. They are aware of why change continues to occur, but haven't been asked to provide input.

Lead with Class

Be malleable. Understand, someone will be the informal leader of the organization. Identify these individuals. Confirm they are on board with the vision of the organization. Lastly, obtain an understanding of who is the formal leader. Their assistance would be greatly appreciated in accomplishing the organization's mission.

Leading with class, my way

The Team

As I *intentionally* walked down the hall, I noticed a housekeeper walking towards me and she quickly said, "Good Morning Dr. Hughes". As we approached each other closer, I smiled and replied, "Good Morning". I then quickly realized that I did not know her name. I wanted to acknowledge her the same way she acknowledged me. So I stopped and turned around and asked her if we had met. She stated we had not, but she knew I was the facility Administrator. That instantly bothered me. Why did I not know her name? So I asked.

Step #4

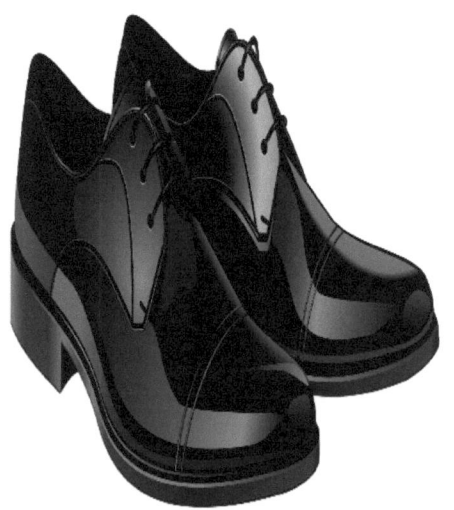

Get to know them.

Should the leader get to know the names of the individuals that do not directly report to them? Absolutely. These persons are directly responsible for carrying out the organization's mission. They are the front line team members.

Step #5

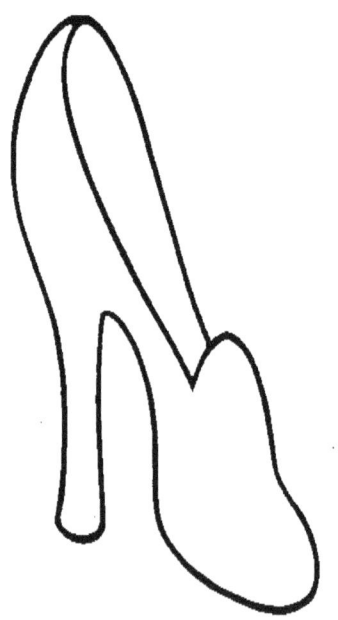

Call them by name.

People like to see and hear their names. Acknowledge them directly, by name, when you see them. Consider recognizing and honoring them publicly. Post their names or photos (birthday, employee of the month, newsletters, etc.).

Step #6

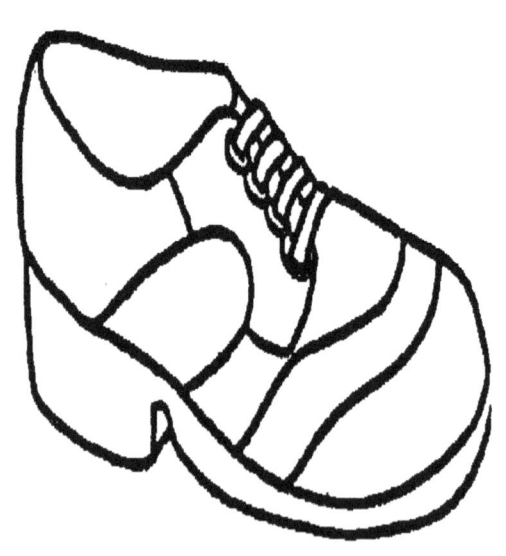

What drives them?

Identify what drives your team members. Are they attending school? Who are their children or grandchildren? Are they newlyweds? When is their work anniversary?

Lead with Class

Be amicable. Understand, people want to feel like they matter. Regardless of their role, they are members of the team. Include them in the decision making. Obtain their input with potential policy changes. Check in with your team members routinely. Consider holding one on one meetings or luncheons where they can openly express themselves.

Leading with class, my way

The Respondent

As I *intentionally* walked to the elevator to meet the emergency medical personnel, my heart begin to beat faster and faster. When the elevator door opened, there he was, the 9 year old asthmatic who was in respiratory distress. As the Emergency Medical Technicians (EMT) were providing a report, I kept my eye on the patient. Although I was listening to the verbal report provided, I wanted to make sure the patient was responding to the treatment that was being administered. The EMTs completed their report and left the room. Then it happened. He coded! Following the process that we were trained to provide, the other nurse and I continued to provide CPR, awaiting the code team. I was the charge nurse and was responsible for contacting the code team? Where were they! Wait….Did I call them?

Step #7

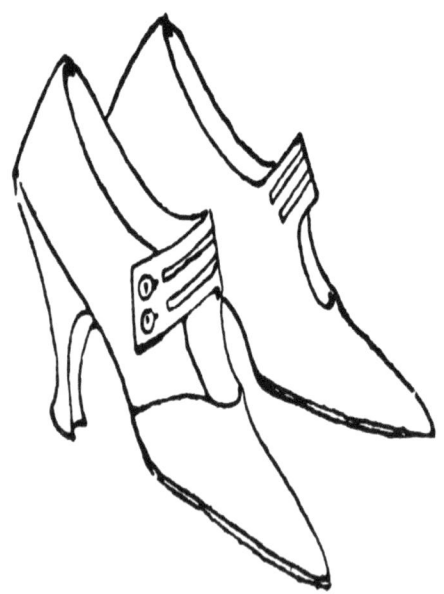

Trust delegation.

Should the leader be responsible for multitasking? The leader is likely to have multiple responsibilities. However, the question is, how many of these responsibilities during a crisis or emergency can be handled by another team member?

Step #8

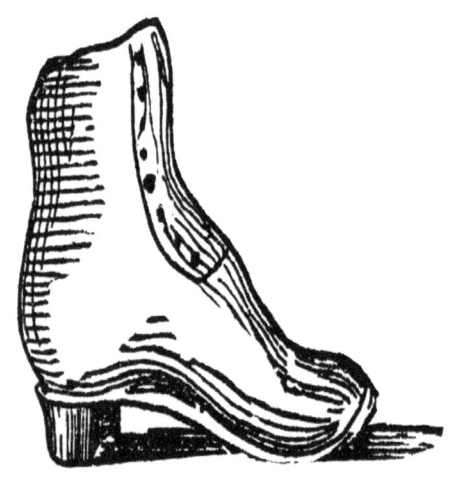

Be transparent.

When we interview individuals we should share the job functions of the position during the interview. Once hired, train the new employee on how to accomplish the job as expected by the organization. This is not school, its training. That means the employee is hired with the required skill. Our role is to ensure training in provided according to the organizations policies, procedures and practices.

Step #9

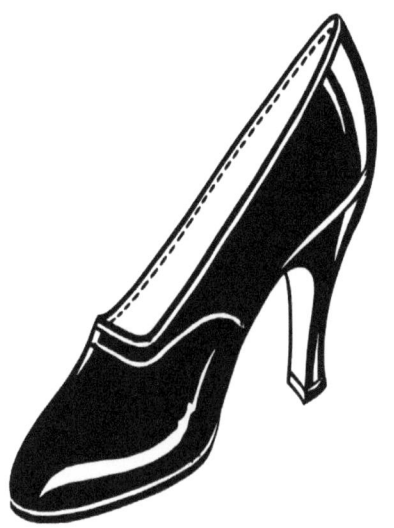

Expect efficiency!

Identify what skills are needed for your team members to be effective. Use scenarios to assist in obtaining a clear understanding of what is expected in various situations.

Lead with Class

Be alert. Understand, people generally want to do their best. We must ensure we equip them with the tools needed to be successful. Identify what skill set is needed to accomplish tasks. Ensure the necessary materials and equipment are available. Consider contingency plans and cross-training to guarantee processes are fully carried through.

Leading with class, my way

The Replacement

As I intentionally walked around the facility, the individuals I encountered had no idea I would be the new Administrator. You see, I would be replacing someone who would be terminated first thing, the next morning. What happened? Did he not follow the organization's policies or was it revenue related (not meeting budget). I wondered had the staff complained about his leadership. What about the patients and families, were they not pleased? The specifics of why the Administrator was being let go was not my biggest concern. I was more concerned with the staff's response to the expeditious change that was about to occur. Were they ready for it (the change)?

Step #10

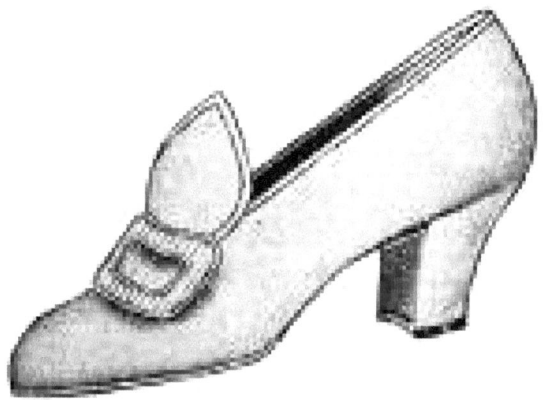

Be a mentor.

Should the leader be in position until they think they are ready to leave the position? The leader should develop a business plan that guides them to accomplishing their endeavors. This plan should include a time line of personal and professional goals. Include the process that will be taken.

Step #11

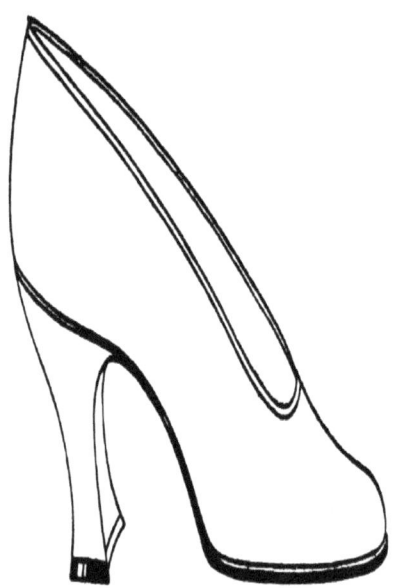

Decompress

When we accept the role of the leader we must be sensitive to the transition that may have taken place, prior to our arrival. There may be resentment, loyalty to the prior leader as well as untruths as why the individual is no longer in the role. It is the new leaders' responsibility to offer the team a time to decompress.

Step #12

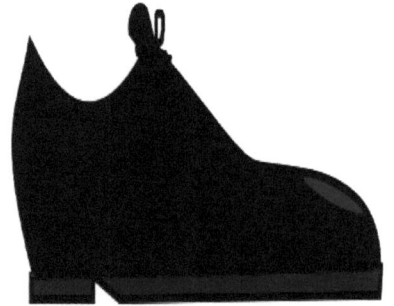

Reset!

Identify what went wrong. Remain transparent to minimize confusion. Keep in mind the reset button is available to be pushed, at the right time.

Lead with Class

Be penetrating. Understand, leaders usually think they are great at what they do. It's not until someone is transparent with us that we realize that we present with the opportunity to do better. To be better. We must remain open to growing. We must also recognize when our season has ended. Consider a succession plan. Pass the torch.

Leading with class, my way

The Line

As I intentionally walked in the front door, I noticed a line of employees standing at my office door awaiting my arrival. I immediately thought, now what happened. One of the nurses stated, "We are glad you are here, we have a problem". As I unlocked the door, the line of employees followed me into the office. After placing my briefcase on the floor, I turned and said, "I haven't had my coffee yet, so I might just say anything"! The four employees looked surprised. I'm not sure why that comment surprised them. Did they not know that I too, had feelings and emotions? Who did they think I really was?

Step #13

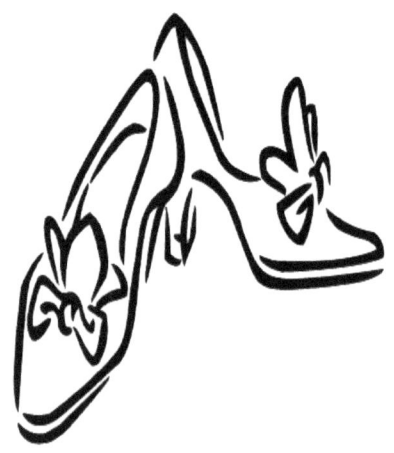

Verify your role.

Should the leader be all things to everyone? It's imperative that the leader recognizes that their role may not be perceived as the 'actual leader". You may be seen as the confidant, the listener, the coach. Recognize and share with the team, the best times, during the day you are listening at your best.

Step #14

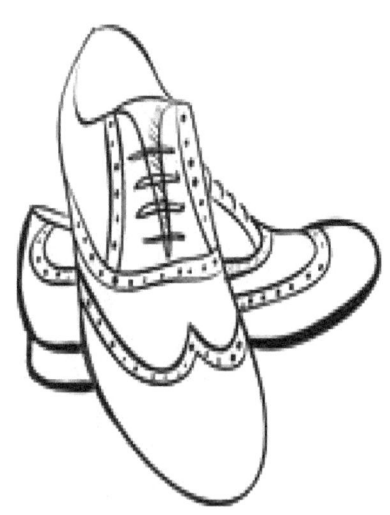

Reflect.

Sometimes repeating what you hear, back to an individual, will allow the person to hear themselves. Hearing yourself provides insight to what the real issue may be.

Step #15

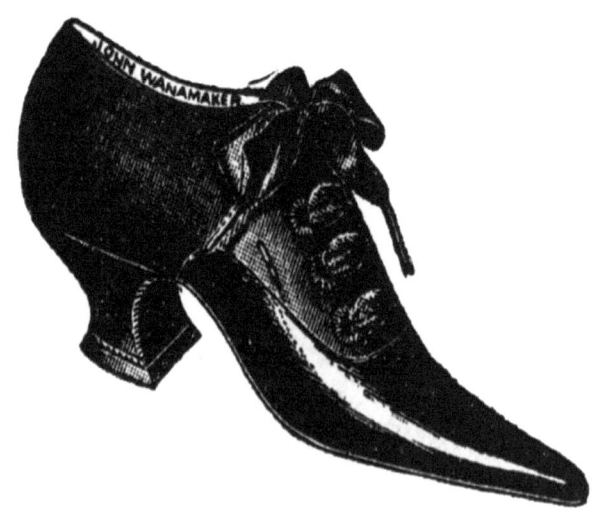

Share

Identify your role. Clarify your personal opinion versus your professional option. Keep in mind what you share may be held within someone for a lifetime. Tread slowly.

Lead with Class

Be a vessel. Understand, the leader is often times seen as all knowing. The employees may find themselves leaning on you for advice (personal and professional). Identify early in the conversation what is the expectation. Consider asking if the question requires action from you or just a listening ear. Always keep in mind your assigned role and theirs.

Leading with class, my way

The Concerned

As I intentionally walked into the patient's room, I instantly noticed the dissatisfied family member's face. I knew the issue had to be big, as they summons me to the room immediately. The daughter continued to voice her dissatisfaction with the care her mother received. As she spoke, tears started to run down my eyes. I thought, could this really be true? Were the employees actually responsible for this? As much to my dismay, the employees validated the accusation.

Step #16

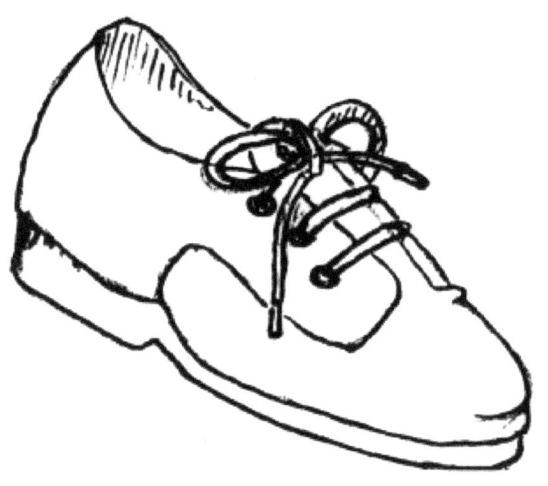

Prevent harm!

Should the leader immediately freeze a bad practice? Yes, specifically if the outcome has the potential of causing harm. During the freeze, a contingent plan would need to be discussed and implemented, until a more permanent process has been identified.

Step #17

Remain calm.

If the potential for harm is apparent, a stand down is necessary. Invite the individuals directly involved. Share the issue in detail and the impact of potential harm it may carry. Discuss how the situation has historically been handled. Review the specifics of how it could have been avoided. Implement a process of education, implementation and evaluation.

Step #18

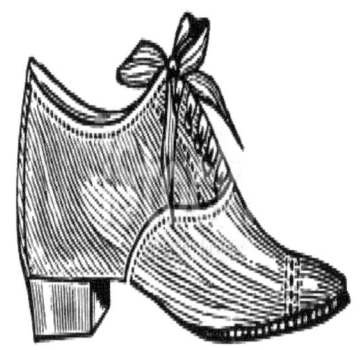

Clarify intentions.

Identify if individuals were intentional in their actions, or was there a misinterpretation of what was expected.

Lead with Class

Be the energy. Understand, the leader consistently evaluates the effectiveness of processes. This evaluation should always include the individuals responsible for implementing the process. In most cases, it will only take a few individuals to develop a new process, when the right people are at the table. Think small, then wide. Move cautiously.

Leading with class, my way

The Moment

As I intentionally walked to my car, headed to the facility to assist the staff with locating a missing patient, I noticed the temperature. It was cold. My next thought, if the patient indeed had left the building, she was also cold. The closer I drove to the facility, my hope was to receive a call that the patient was found. I did not receive the call. When I pulled up to my assigned parking spot, and stepped out of my car, the search and rescue dog, sniffed at my feet. It was at that moment I knew, this was going to be unforgettable.

Step #19

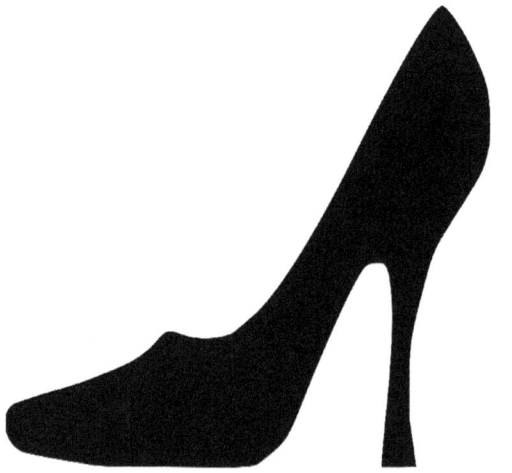

Provide refuge.

Should the leader ultimately be held responsible for the safety and security of the customers and staff? Absolutely.

Step #20

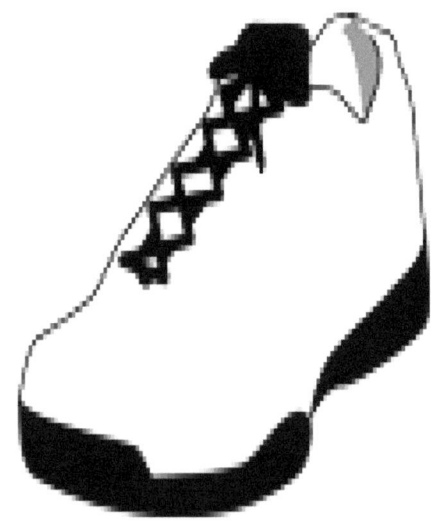

Round daily.

In every industry, safety should take priority over ALL things. Daily safety rounds must be a common practice. The best practice is to have the rounds conducted by the individuals who do not routine work in the department.

Step #21

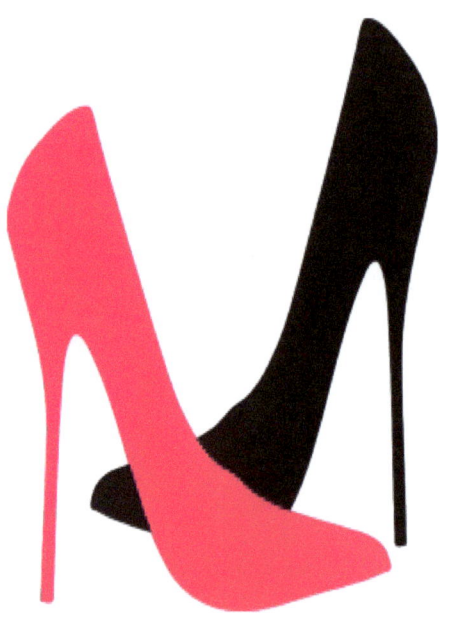

Identify risk!

Identify safety risks through listening and observing, then discussing.

Lead with Class

Be a shield. Understand, the leader is ultimately responsible for ensuring the employees and customers are safe. This goes far beyond the wet floor signs. Safety discussions should start during the interview process. The individuals you employ, should know early in the hiring process, the emphasis you place on safety.

Leading with class, my way

*The intentional leader who has **CLASS** should be a blessing regardless of obstacles!*

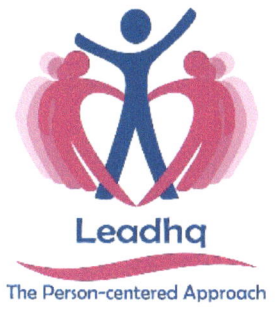

A LEADERSHIP AND HEALTHCARE QUALITY GIFTBOOK

www.ingramcontent.com/pod-product-compliance
Lightning Source LLC
Chambersburg PA
CBHW040226220526
45473CB00001B/143